I0702233

Herbal Remedies for Flat Tummy

The Natural Medicine Solutions to Reduce Belly Fat, Improve Digestion, and Relieve Bloating

NatureCures Press

Copyright © 2024 NatureCures Press

All rights reserved. No part of this publication may be reproduced, stored in a retrieval system, or transmitted in any form or by any means, electronic, mechanical, photocopying, recording, or otherwise, without the prior written permission of the author.

Table of Contents

Introduction

Welcome to Herbal Remedies for Flat Tummy, a comprehensive guide dedicated to exploring the natural medicine solutions for reducing belly fat, improving digestion, and relieving bloating. In this guide, we will delve into the intricate relationship between herbs and a healthy midsection, aiming to provide you with valuable insights on achieving and maintaining a flat tummy through herbal remedies.

A healthy midsection is not only aesthetically pleasing but is also crucial for overall well-being. Belly fat, often considered stubborn, can pose significant health risks. Understanding the nuances of belly fat is the first step towards its effective reduction. We'll explore the various types of belly fat and the factors that contribute to its accumulation, establishing a foundational understanding of the science behind it.

Beyond the cosmetic aspect, excess abdominal fat can lead to health issues such as cardiovascular diseases and diabetes. This chapter aims to shed light on the health implications of belly fat, emphasizing the importance of adopting holistic approaches for its reduction.

How Herbal Remedies Can Aid in Achieving a Flat Tummy

Herbs have been integral to traditional medicine systems for centuries, offering a wealth of natural remedies. In the context of achieving a flat tummy, understanding how herbs can play a pivotal role is essential. We will discuss the science behind herbal remedies, exploring how certain herbs support digestion, boost metabolism, and contribute to weight loss.

Herbs possess a range of properties that can aid in addressing the root causes of belly fat, whether it's sluggish digestion, hormonal imbalances, or inflammation. This chapter will provide a detailed examination of the specific ways in which herbal remedies interact with the body to promote a healthier midsection.

Chapter 1

The Science Behind Belly Fat

Belly fat, scientifically known as visceral fat, is a complex and dynamic aspect of human physiology that extends beyond its visual manifestation. Understanding the science behind belly fat is pivotal in formulating effective strategies for its reduction and overall health improvement.

Exploring the Different Types of Belly Fat

Belly fat, scientifically known as visceral fat, is a complex and dynamic aspect of human physiology that extends beyond its visual manifestation. Understanding the science behind belly fat is pivotal in formulating effective strategies for its reduction and overall health improvement.

Visceral fat is not a uniform entity; rather, it consists of different types with unique characteristics and implications for health. Subcutaneous fat, the adipose tissue beneath the skin, differs from visceral fat, which surrounds internal organs. While subcutaneous fat has functions such as insulation and energy storage, visceral fat poses more significant health risks due to its proximity to vital organs.

Within the realm of visceral fat, there are distinct compartments. Some individuals may predominantly accumulate fat around the liver, referred to as hepatic fat, while others may have a higher concentration around the intestines, known as omentum fat. Understanding these nuances is crucial as the distribution of fat can influence health outcomes differently.

Research indicates that visceral fat is metabolically active, producing hormones and cytokines that can impact various bodily functions. For instance, it secretes adiponectin, a hormone associated with insulin sensitivity, but also releases inflammatory substances. This dynamic interaction underscores the need for a nuanced approach when addressing different types of belly fat.

Moreover, the varying distribution of fat in different individuals can be influenced by genetic factors.

Understanding these genetic predispositions sheds light on why some people may be more prone to accumulating visceral fat than others. This exploration into the different types of belly fat provides a foundational understanding of the intricacies involved, paving the way for targeted approaches to its reduction.

Understanding the Factors Contributing to Belly Fat Accumulation

The accumulation of belly fat is a multifaceted phenomenon influenced by a myriad of factors that extend beyond mere caloric imbalance. Genetic predisposition, lifestyle choices, hormonal fluctuations, and age-related changes all play significant roles in the development of excess abdominal fat.

Genetics, in particular, can exert a substantial influence on an individual's propensity to accumulate belly fat. Research has identified specific genetic markers associated with abdominal obesity, shedding light on why some individuals may be more predisposed to store fat around the midsection. Acknowledging these genetic factors is crucial in developing personalized strategies for belly fat reduction.

Lifestyle choices, encompassing dietary habits and levels of physical activity, are pivotal contributors to belly fat accumulation. A diet rich in refined sugars and saturated fats, coupled with a sedentary lifestyle, creates a conducive environment for fat storage, especially around the abdominal region. Understanding the impact of these lifestyle choices underscores the importance of comprehensive interventions that address both diet and exercise patterns.

Hormonal fluctuations play a significant role in belly fat accumulation, with imbalances in insulin and cortisol levels being key contributors. Insulin resistance, often associated with a diet high in processed foods, can lead to increased fat storage around the abdomen. Elevated cortisol levels, a response to chronic stress, can further exacerbate this issue by promoting fat deposition in the abdominal area.

Age-related changes in metabolism also contribute to belly fat accumulation. As individuals age, there tends to be a decline in muscle mass, leading to a decrease in basal metabolic rate. This makes it easier to gain weight, especially around the abdominal area, and more challenging to lose it. Understanding the impact of age on metabolism provides insights into the challenges that may arise in addressing belly fat as individuals grow older.

In essence, comprehending the various factors contributing to belly fat accumulation is integral to developing effective and targeted strategies for its reduction. By acknowledging the roles of genetics, lifestyle choices, hormonal imbalances, and age-related changes, individuals can tailor their approaches to address the specific factors influencing their abdominal fat.

Importance of a Holistic Approach to Belly Fat Reduction

Addressing belly fat reduction holistically involves recognizing the interconnected nature of various factors influencing its accumulation and adopting comprehensive lifestyle changes. Focusing solely on isolated interventions, such as crash diets or specific exercises, often yields limited success and fails to address the underlying issues contributing to belly fat accumulation.

A holistic approach considers the multifaceted aspects of an individual's life that contribute to belly fat accumulation, emphasizing the integration of dietary modifications, regular physical activity, stress management, and adequate sleep. This approach recognizes that effective belly fat reduction requires a combination of interventions that collectively address the root causes.

Diet plays a pivotal role in any holistic approach to belly fat reduction. Emphasizing whole foods, incorporating a variety of nutrient-dense fruits and vegetables, and opting for lean protein sources contribute to a balanced and supportive diet. The inclusion of dietary fiber aids in digestion and promotes a feeling of fullness, reducing the likelihood of overeating.

Regular physical activity is a cornerstone of holistic belly fat reduction. Both aerobic exercises, such as running or swimming, and strength training exercises contribute to calorie burning and metabolic enhancement. Additionally, strength training helps build muscle mass, which can positively impact metabolism and contribute to the loss of visceral fat.

Stress management is often underestimated but is a crucial component of holistic belly fat reduction. Chronic stress can lead to elevated cortisol levels, promoting the storage of fat, especially around the abdominal area. Incorporating stress-reducing activities, such as meditation, yoga, or mindfulness practices, helps regulate cortisol levels and mitigate the impact of stress on belly fat accumulation.

Adequate sleep is a fundamental but often overlooked aspect of a holistic approach to belly fat reduction. Sleep influences hormonal balance, particularly the regulation of appetite hormones like leptin and ghrelin. Sleep deprivation can disrupt these hormones, leading to increased cravings and overeating, contributing to belly fat accumulation.

Chapter 2

Herbs for Digestive Health

Herbs have been revered for centuries for their therapeutic properties, and when it comes to digestive health, their role is particularly noteworthy.

Overview of Herbs Supporting Digestion

Herbs have long been recognized for their potential to promote digestive health. A myriad of herbs boasts properties that aid in the digestion process, addressing common issues such as bloating, indigestion, and sluggish digestion. One notable group of digestive herbs includes carminatives, which are known for their ability to ease gas and bloating.

Among the prominent digestive herbs is peppermint, celebrated for its calming effect on the gastrointestinal tract. Peppermint's active compound, menthol, helps relax the muscles of the gastrointestinal tract, alleviating symptoms of indigestion. Additionally, ginger, with its anti-inflammatory and anti-nausea properties, is known to support digestion by promoting the flow of digestive juices.

Fennel, an aromatic herb with a mild licorice flavor, is another digestive powerhouse. Its carminative properties help soothe the digestive tract and reduce bloating. Chamomile, often consumed as a calming tea, possesses anti-inflammatory properties that contribute to its digestive benefits. These herbs, among others, collectively contribute to a holistic approach to digestive health.

Understanding the mechanisms by which these herbs support digestion provides insights into their therapeutic applications. From promoting the secretion of digestive enzymes to relaxing the muscles of the digestive tract, these herbs act synergistically to enhance overall digestive function. This overview sets the stage for a deeper exploration into the specific ways in which herbs can be harnessed for digestive well-being.

Herbal Teas for Improved Digestion

Herbal teas stand out as a delightful and accessible means of incorporating digestive herbs into one's routine while simultaneously providing a comforting and soothing experience. Various herbal teas have been revered for their digestive benefits, offering a natural and enjoyable way to support the intricate processes of digestion.

Peppermint tea, derived from the leaves of the peppermint plant, is widely celebrated for its ability to alleviate digestive discomfort. The menthol in peppermint not only relaxes the muscles of the gastrointestinal tract but also helps relieve symptoms of irritable bowel syndrome (IBS). Sipping on a warm cup of peppermint tea after a meal can provide a gentle yet effective digestive boost.

Chamomile tea, derived from the flowers of the chamomile plant, is known for its anti-inflammatory and calming properties. Beyond promoting relaxation and reducing stress, chamomile tea can ease indigestion and bloating. Its gentle nature makes it a suitable choice for those with sensitive digestive systems.

Ginger tea, crafted from the rhizome of the ginger plant, is a zesty and invigorating option for supporting digestion. Gingerol, the active compound in ginger, possesses anti-inflammatory and anti-nausea properties. Ginger tea can stimulate the digestive process, making it particularly beneficial for those experiencing sluggish digestion.

Fennel tea, brewed from fennel seeds, is another herbal infusion with notable digestive benefits. Its carminative properties help alleviate bloating and gas, making it a go-to choice for those seeking digestive comfort. The mildly sweet and aromatic flavor of fennel tea adds a delightful touch to the overall experience.

The act of sipping herbal teas itself contributes to digestive well-being. The warmth of the tea can have a soothing effect on the digestive tract, promoting relaxation and aiding in the overall digestion process. The ritualistic aspect of enjoying a cup of herbal tea also adds a mindful element to the experience, encouraging individuals to savor the moment and be present with their digestive processes.

Incorporating Digestive Herbs into Daily Routine

Embracing digestive herbs in daily routines extends beyond the realm of teas, offering diverse and creative ways to harness their benefits. From culinary applications to herbal supplements, there are numerous avenues for individuals to seamlessly integrate digestive herbs into their lifestyles.

In the realm of culinary exploration, herbs like basil, cilantro, and dill not only enhance the flavor profiles of dishes but also contribute to digestive health. These herbs possess carminative properties, aiding in the digestion of fats and promoting overall digestive comfort. Incorporating fresh herbs into salads, soups, and various dishes not only elevates culinary experiences but also adds a nutritional and digestive boost.

For those seeking convenience, herbal supplements provide a concentrated and potent form of digestive support. Digestive enzyme supplements, often containing herbs like ginger and peppermint, can assist the body in breaking down and absorbing nutrients more efficiently. These supplements are particularly beneficial for individuals with conditions such as pancreatic insufficiency or other digestive disorders.

Essential oils extracted from digestive herbs open up yet another avenue for daily use. Adding a drop of peppermint essential oil to a glass of water or inhaling its aroma can offer quick relief from indigestion. Similarly, ginger essential oil, known for its warming and soothing properties, can be diluted and applied topically to the abdomen for digestive comfort.

In the context of holistic well-being, incorporating mindfulness practices into daily routines complements the digestive benefits of herbs. Practices such as mindful eating, where individuals savor each bite and pay attention to the sensory experience of food, contribute to optimal digestion. Mindful practices not only foster a deeper connection with the act of eating but also promote a relaxed state conducive to digestive processes.

Chapter 3

Herbal Remedies for Belly Fat Reduction

Role of Herbs in Metabolism Boosting

The intricate relationship between herbs and metabolism has long been acknowledged, and in the pursuit of belly fat reduction, understanding the role of herbs in metabolism boosting becomes pivotal. Metabolism, the complex set of biochemical processes that convert food into energy, plays a central role in determining how efficiently the body utilizes calories. Herbs, with their diverse array of bioactive compounds, can influence and enhance metabolic functions.

Several herbs are renowned for their ability to stimulate metabolic rate and promote calorie expenditure. One such herb is green tea, celebrated for its high content of catechins, particularly epigallocatechin gallate (EGCG). Research suggests that EGCG can elevate metabolism, increasing the rate at which the body burns calories. Incorporating green tea into one's routine, whether through traditional brewing or as a supplement, can be a strategic move in supporting metabolic processes.

Cayenne pepper, known for its spicy kick, contains capsaicin, a compound linked to metabolism-boosting effects. Capsaicin has been found to increase thermogenesis, where the body generates heat and expends energy. By incorporating cayenne pepper into meals or opting for supplements, individuals may harness its metabolism-boosting properties to aid in belly fat reduction.

Ginger, beyond its digestive benefits, has also been associated with a positive impact on metabolism. Gingerol, the active compound in ginger, exhibits thermogenic properties, contributing to increased calorie burning. Whether consumed in tea, added to dishes, or taken as a supplement, ginger stands as a versatile herb that can support metabolic functions.

Moreover, herbs like cinnamon have been linked to improved insulin sensitivity, influencing how the body processes sugars and manages blood glucose levels. By enhancing insulin sensitivity, cinnamon may contribute to better metabolic regulation, potentially influencing the body's ability to store and utilize fats. Including cinnamon in diets, whether in recipes or sprinkled over beverages, offers a flavorful and metabolic-boosting option.

The role of herbs in metabolism boosting extends beyond individual components; it encompasses the synergy of various compounds working in concert. Herbs provide a holistic approach to metabolism, influencing factors such as thermogenesis, insulin sensitivity, and nutrient partitioning. Understanding the specific mechanisms by which herbs contribute to metabolic functions empowers individuals in crafting effective strategies for belly fat reduction.

Herbal Supplements to Aid Weight Loss

The realm of weight loss has seen a surge in interest surrounding herbal supplements, as individuals seek natural and holistic approaches to shedding excess pounds. Herbal supplements, derived from a variety of plants and botanicals, offer a diverse range of compounds that can potentially support weight loss efforts. Understanding the role of herbal supplements in aiding weight loss involves exploring their mechanisms, potential benefits, and considerations for safe and effective use.

One notable herbal supplement that has gained widespread attention is Garcinia Cambogia. Extracted from the rind of the Garcinia Cambogia fruit, this supplement contains hydroxycitric acid (HCA), believed to inhibit an enzyme that plays a role in fat storage. Some studies suggest that Garcinia Cambogia may contribute to modest weight loss when combined with a healthy diet and exercise. However, it's crucial to note that individual responses to this supplement can vary, and its efficacy remains a topic of ongoing research.

Green coffee bean extract is another herbal supplement that has garnered interest in the weight loss realm. Green coffee beans, before they undergo the roasting process, contain chlorogenic acid, believed to have potential effects on metabolism and fat absorption. While some studies suggest a modest reduction in body weight with green coffee bean extract, more research is needed to fully understand its long-term effects and optimal usage.

Certain herbs, such as forskolin, derived from the roots of the Indian Coleus plant, have been investigated for their potential impact on weight loss. Forskolin is believed to stimulate the production of cAMP, a molecule that plays a role in cellular signaling. Some studies suggest that forskolin may help promote the breakdown of stored fats. However, the research on forskolin is still in its early stages, and more evidence is needed to establish its efficacy and safety for weight loss.

In addition to specific herbal extracts, herbal blends formulated for weight loss have become prevalent in the market. These blends often combine a variety of herbs known for their potential impact on metabolism, appetite regulation, and fat metabolism. Ingredients such as green tea extract, garcinia cambogia, and cayenne pepper may be combined in these formulations to create a synergistic effect, aiming to address multiple aspects of weight loss.

It's important to approach herbal supplements for weight loss with a discerning mindset. While some herbs may show promise in supporting weight loss goals, they are not a magic solution. Weight loss remains a complex interplay of various factors, including diet, physical activity, and overall lifestyle. Herbal supplements should complement a holistic approach to weight management rather than serve as a standalone solution.

Moreover, the quality and purity of herbal supplements play a crucial role in their effectiveness and safety. Choosing reputable brands, consulting with healthcare professionals, and being aware of potential side effects are essential considerations when incorporating herbal supplements into one's weight loss regimen. Like any supplement, herbal formulations should be approached with caution, particularly for individuals with underlying health conditions or those taking medications.

Creating Herbal Blends for Belly Fat Reduction

The art of herbalism extends beyond individual herbs and supplements; it encompasses the harmonious blending of diverse botanicals to create herbal combinations tailored for specific purposes. In the context of belly fat reduction, crafting herbal blends becomes a nuanced and creative endeavor. This chapter explores the principles behind creating herbal blends for targeted fat reduction, the synergy of key herbs, and practical tips for incorporating these blends into daily routines.

Principles Behind Creating Herbal Blends

Creating effective herbal blends for belly fat reduction involves a thoughtful consideration of the properties and synergies of individual herbs. Each herb contributes unique compounds and benefits, and when combined strategically, they can create a blend that addresses multiple aspects of fat metabolism and overall well-being.

One fundamental principle is understanding the thermogenic properties of certain herbs. Herbs like cayenne pepper and ginger, known for their ability to generate heat in the body, can contribute to increased calorie expenditure. Incorporating these thermogenic herbs into blends can support the body in burning additional calories, potentially aiding in the reduction of stored fat.

Another principle revolves around herbs that support digestion and metabolic functions. Herbs like dandelion, fennel, and peppermint can assist in optimizing digestion, ensuring that nutrients are effectively absorbed and utilized by the body. A well-functioning digestive system is essential for overall health and plays a crucial role in the body's ability to manage weight.

Furthermore, incorporating herbs with adaptogenic properties into blends can be beneficial. Adaptogens, such as rhodiola and holy basil, help the body adapt to stress and maintain balance. Stress management is a crucial aspect of belly fat reduction, as chronic stress can contribute to the accumulation of visceral fat. Blends that include adaptogenic herbs aim to promote overall well-being and resilience in the face of stressors.

Understanding the flavor profiles of herbs is also key in creating blends that are enjoyable and palatable. Blending bitter herbs like dandelion with aromatic and soothing herbs like chamomile can result in a well-rounded flavor profile that not only supports digestion but also makes the herbal blend more appealing to the palate.

Synergy of Key Herbs in Belly Fat Reduction Blends

Synergy is the magic that happens when various herbs work together, enhancing each other's properties and creating a more potent effect than individual herbs alone. In the context of belly fat reduction, certain key herbs exhibit remarkable synergy when combined thoughtfully.

Green tea, renowned for its metabolism-boosting properties, can be a cornerstone of belly fat reduction blends. Its high catechin content, particularly EGCG, complements the thermogenic effects of herbs like cayenne pepper. Blending green tea with peppermint and ginger not only creates a flavorful infusion but also combines herbs that support digestion and enhance the overall metabolic impact of the blend.

Dandelion and fennel, both known for their digestive benefits, synergize well in belly fat reduction blends. Dandelion's bitter compounds stimulate digestion and liver function, while fennel's carminative properties help alleviate bloating. Combining these herbs with a touch of lemon balm or mint can result in a refreshing blend that supports digestive comfort.

Turmeric, with its active compound curcumin, is celebrated for its anti-inflammatory properties. Including turmeric in belly fat reduction blends contributes not only to reducing inflammation but also to overall metabolic health. Pairing turmeric with black pepper, which enhances the absorption of curcumin, creates a dynamic duo in herbal blends.

Cinnamon, known for its potential to improve insulin sensitivity, can complement the effects of herbs like gymnema sylvestre in blends aimed at balancing blood sugar levels. Gymnema sylvestre is an herb traditionally used to support healthy glucose metabolism. Blending these herbs with the warming notes of ginger and a hint of licorice creates a well-balanced and supportive herbal infusion.

Holy basil, an adaptogenic herb, can enhance the stress-relieving properties of blends aimed at belly fat reduction. Combining holy basil with calming herbs like chamomile or lavender creates a blend that not only supports stress management but also contributes to overall well-being.

Practical Tips for Incorporating Herbal Blends into Daily Routines

Creating herbal blends for belly fat reduction is not only about selecting the right herbs but also about seamlessly integrating these blends into daily routines. Practicality and consistency are key in realizing the potential benefits of herbal infusions. Here are some practical tips for incorporating herbal blends into daily life:

Morning Rituals: Start the day with a metabolism-boosting herbal blend. A combination of green tea, cayenne pepper, and a touch of lemon can create an invigorating infusion to kickstart the metabolism. Enjoy it as part of your morning rituals to set a positive tone for the day.

Midday Digestive Support: Consider a midday herbal blend that supports digestion and alleviates any bloating or discomfort. Dandelion, fennel, and peppermint make an excellent trio for a refreshing and digestive-friendly infusion. Sip on it after meals to aid digestion.

Afternoon Pick-Me-Up: Combat afternoon fatigue and cravings with a blend that includes adaptogenic herbs like holy basil or rhodiola. Adding a touch of cinnamon can contribute to blood sugar balance. This afternoon pick-me-up can provide a natural energy boost and help manage stress.

Evening Relaxation: Wind down in the evening with a calming herbal blend. Chamomile, lavender, and turmeric create a soothing infusion that not only promotes relaxation but also supports anti-inflammatory and metabolic functions. Incorporate this blend into your evening routine to signal the body that it's time to unwind.

Consistency is Key: To experience the potential benefits of herbal blends for belly fat reduction, consistency is crucial. Make herbal infusions a regular part of your routine, adjusting the blends based on your preferences and needs. Whether it's a warm cup in the morning or a refreshing iced infusion in the afternoon, find what works best for you.

Experiment and Personalize: Herbalism is an art, and personal preferences play a significant role. Feel free to experiment with different herbs, ratios, and flavor combinations to tailor blends to your liking. Consider consulting with herbalists or healthcare professionals for personalized guidance based on your health goals and individual needs.

Chapter 4

Alleviating Bloating Naturally

Understanding the Causes of Bloating

Bloating, a common and often uncomfortable sensation, can arise from a variety of factors. Understanding the causes of bloating is essential for implementing effective strategies to alleviate this condition naturally. One primary contributor to bloating is the accumulation of gas in the digestive system. This can occur due to the fermentation of undigested food in the colon, leading to the production of gases such as methane and hydrogen. Additionally, swallowing air while eating or drinking, often unintentionally, contributes to the presence of gas in the digestive tract.

Certain foods are notorious for causing bloating, with cruciferous vegetables, beans, and carbonated beverages being notable culprits. These foods contain complex carbohydrates and fibers that can be challenging to digest fully, leading to gas production. Individuals with lactose intolerance may experience bloating when consuming dairy products, as their bodies lack the enzyme needed to break down lactose.

Digestive disorders such as irritable bowel syndrome (IBS) and inflammatory bowel disease (IBD) can also contribute to chronic bloating. In IBS, irregular contractions of the intestinal muscles can lead to gas accumulation and bloating. In IBD, inflammation of the digestive tract may cause changes in bowel habits and abdominal discomfort, including bloating.

Furthermore, hormonal fluctuations, particularly in women during menstruation or pregnancy, can influence water retention and contribute to bloating. Stress, a ubiquitous factor in modern lifestyles, can impact digestion by altering the movement of the digestive tract and promoting bloating. Understanding the diverse factors that contribute to bloating sets the stage for exploring natural remedies that target specific causes.

Herbs for Bloating Relief

Herbs have long been valued for their ability to provide natural relief from various ailments, and bloating is no exception. Incorporating specific herbs into one's routine can help address the underlying causes of bloating and promote digestive comfort.

Peppermint, with its menthol compound, stands out as a potent herb for bloating relief. It has been shown to relax the muscles of the gastrointestinal tract, reducing spasms and alleviating symptoms of indigestion and bloating. Peppermint tea, in particular, is a popular and soothing way to harness the digestive benefits of this herb.

Ginger, known for its anti-inflammatory and digestive properties, is another herbal ally in bloating relief. Ginger can help stimulate the digestive process, alleviate gas, and reduce bloating. Whether consumed in tea, added to meals, or taken in supplement form, ginger offers a versatile and effective option for promoting digestive well-being.

Fennel, an aromatic herb with a mild licorice flavor, has been traditionally used to ease digestive discomfort and bloating. Fennel seeds contain compounds with carminative properties, helping to relax the digestive tract and reduce gas. Fennel tea, brewed from the seeds, is a gentle and flavorful remedy for bloating.

Chamomile, known for its calming and anti-inflammatory effects, can contribute to bloating relief by soothing the digestive system. Chamomile tea, enjoyed warm or as an iced infusion, provides not only a delightful beverage but also a natural remedy for digestive discomfort.

Cinnamon, with its sweet and warming flavor, has been associated with reducing bloating by promoting healthy digestion. Cinnamon can help regulate blood sugar levels, potentially preventing spikes and crashes that contribute to bloating. Incorporating cinnamon into herbal blends or sprinkling it over foods can be an enjoyable way to benefit from its digestive support.

These herbs, among others, offer a holistic approach to bloating relief by addressing various factors contributing to digestive discomfort. Their natural properties provide gentle yet effective solutions, making them suitable for regular use as part of a well-rounded approach to digestive health.

Herbal Infusions for a Flatter Stomach

Herbal infusions, crafted from a combination of bloating-relief herbs, offer a flavorful and hydrating way to alleviate bloating and promote a flatter stomach. Creating herbal infusions involves steeping herbs in hot water, allowing their beneficial compounds to be released and infused into the liquid. Here are some herbal infusions that can contribute to a flatter stomach:

- **Peppermint and Ginger Infusion:** Combining peppermint and ginger in an herbal infusion creates a dynamic blend that targets bloating from multiple angles. Peppermint helps relax the muscles of the digestive tract, while ginger stimulates digestion and alleviates gas. The combination of these herbs provides a refreshing and effective infusion for digestive comfort.

- **Fennel and Chamomile Infusion:** Blending fennel seeds with chamomile flowers creates a soothing infusion that calms the digestive system and reduces bloating. Fennel's carminative properties complement the anti-inflammatory effects of chamomile, making this infusion an excellent choice for promoting relaxation and digestive well-being.

- **Cinnamon and Cardamom Infusion:** Infusing cinnamon and cardamom creates a warm and aromatic blend that not only delights the senses but also supports digestive health. Cinnamon's ability to regulate blood sugar levels, coupled with cardamom's carminative properties, makes this infusion a flavorful option for those seeking a natural remedy for bloating.

- **Lemon Balm and Peppermint Infusion:** Lemon balm, known for its calming effects, combines harmoniously with peppermint to create an infusion that eases digestive discomfort and promotes relaxation. This infusion can be enjoyed hot or cold, making it a versatile choice for various preferences and occasions.

- **Ginger and Turmeric Infusion:** Infusing ginger and turmeric brings together two potent herbs with anti-inflammatory properties. This blend not only aids in reducing bloating but also provides additional support for overall digestive and metabolic health. The warming notes of ginger complement the earthy flavor of turmeric, creating a well-balanced and beneficial infusion.

Incorporating herbal infusions into daily routines offers a convenient and enjoyable way to support digestive health. These infusions can be enjoyed throughout the day, whether as a morning ritual, an afternoon pick-me-up, or a soothing evening beverage. Experimenting with different herb combinations and finding the flavors that resonate with individual preferences adds a creative dimension to the journey toward a flatter stomach.

Chapter 5

Lifestyle Changes for a Flat Tummy

Achieving a flat tummy extends beyond specific remedies or herbal solutions; it involves embracing holistic lifestyle changes that contribute to overall well-being.

Importance of Physical Activity

Physical activity stands as a cornerstone in the pursuit of a flat tummy and overall health. Regular exercise not only burns calories but also plays a crucial role in toning abdominal muscles and reducing visceral fat—the type of fat that accumulates around internal organs and contributes to the appearance of a protruding belly.

Engaging in cardiovascular exercises, such as running, brisk walking, or cycling, elevates the heart rate and enhances calorie expenditure. These activities not only contribute to overall weight loss but also specifically target the reduction of abdominal fat. Moreover, incorporating strength training exercises, like planks, squats, and core workouts, strengthens the abdominal muscles, providing a firmer and more toned midsection.

The impact of physical activity extends beyond the visible changes in body composition. Exercise stimulates the release of endorphins, often referred to as "feel-good" hormones, which contribute to improved mood and reduced stress. This psychological benefit is integral to a holistic approach to health, as mental well-being is intertwined with physical well-being.

Consistency is key when it comes to physical activity. Establishing a routine that includes a mix of cardiovascular and strength training exercises, tailored to individual fitness levels and preferences, ensures a sustainable and effective approach. Whether it's a daily jog, a fitness class, or home workouts, finding enjoyable and varied forms of exercise contributes not only to a flat tummy but also to overall vitality.

Beyond structured exercise, incorporating movement into daily life is equally important.

Simple habits like taking the stairs, walking instead of driving for short distances, or stretching during breaks can collectively contribute to increased physical activity. Adopting a lifestyle that prioritizes movement supports the body's natural processes and complements other efforts for a flat tummy.

Balancing Diet for Belly Fat Reduction

Diet plays a pivotal role in the quest for a flat tummy, and the emphasis goes beyond mere calorie counting. Adopting a balanced and nourishing diet contributes to sustainable weight management and the reduction of abdominal fat. Here are key considerations for crafting a diet conducive to belly fat reduction:

- **Emphasize Whole Foods:** Incorporating whole, nutrient-dense foods into the diet provides essential vitamins, minerals, and fiber. Fruits, vegetables, whole grains, lean proteins, and healthy fats contribute to satiety and support overall health. Fiber, in particular, aids in digestion and helps prevent constipation, reducing the likelihood of bloating.

- **Mindful Eating:** Practicing mindful eating involves paying attention to hunger and fullness cues, savoring the flavors of food, and avoiding distractions during meals. This approach fosters a healthy relationship with food, promotes better digestion, and prevents overeating.

- **Portion Control:** While the quality of food is crucial, managing portion sizes is equally important. Being mindful of portion control helps regulate calorie intake and prevents excessive consumption. Utilizing smaller plates, measuring portions, and paying attention to hunger signals contribute to effective portion control.

- **Hydration:** Staying well-hydrated is a simple yet powerful aspect of a balanced diet. Water supports digestion, helps maintain a feeling of fullness, and contributes to overall metabolic functions. Opting for water as the primary beverage choice over sugary drinks or excessive caffeine supports both hydration and belly fat reduction.

- **Limit Added Sugars and Processed Foods:** Excessive consumption of added sugars and highly processed foods contributes to inflammation and weight gain, particularly in the abdominal region. Minimizing the intake of sugary snacks, sodas, and processed foods helps create a diet focused on nutrient-dense, whole foods.

- **Include Healthy Fats:** Incorporating sources of healthy fats, such as avocados, nuts, seeds, and olive oil, supports overall health and satiety. Healthy fats contribute to a feeling of fullness and provide a steady source of energy, reducing the likelihood of overeating.

Adopting a balanced diet is not about strict restrictions but rather about making sustainable and informed choices that align with individual preferences and health goals. Working with a registered dietitian or nutrition professional can provide personalized guidance based on individual needs and ensure a well-rounded approach to belly fat reduction.

Stress Management for a Healthy Midsection

Stress, a ubiquitous aspect of modern life, significantly influences both mental and physical well-being, including the appearance of the midsection. Chronic stress triggers the release of cortisol, a hormone associated with the body's "fight or flight" response. Elevated cortisol levels, over time, contribute to the accumulation of visceral fat, particularly around the abdominal area.

Managing stress is therefore a vital component of cultivating a healthy midsection. Incorporating stress-reducing practices into daily life contributes not only to belly fat reduction but also to overall mental and emotional well-being. Here are effective strategies for stress management:

- **Mindfulness and Meditation:** Mindfulness practices, including meditation and deep-breathing exercises, promote relaxation and help mitigate the impact of stress on the body. These practices encourage present-moment awareness, fostering a sense of calm and reducing cortisol levels.

- **Regular Physical Activity:** Exercise, beyond its physical benefits, serves as a powerful tool for stress management. Engaging in regular physical activity helps release endorphins, the body's natural stress relievers. Whether it's a brisk walk, a yoga session, or a workout routine, physical activity contributes to a balanced and resilient response to stress.

- **Adequate Sleep:** Prioritizing quality sleep is fundamental to stress management. Lack of sleep can disrupt hormonal balance, including cortisol regulation, leading to increased stress levels. Establishing consistent sleep patterns and creating a conducive sleep environment contribute to overall well-being.

- **Social Connection:** Building and maintaining social connections provide emotional support and serve as a buffer against stress. Whether through friendships, family relationships, or community involvement, fostering social connections contributes to a sense of belonging and resilience in the face of stressors.

- **Time Management and Prioritization:** Effective time management and setting realistic priorities contribute to stress reduction. Breaking tasks into manageable steps, setting boundaries, and learning to say no when necessary prevent overwhelming stress and create a more balanced lifestyle.

- **Hobbies and Relaxation Activities:** Engaging in hobbies and activities that bring joy and relaxation is an essential aspect of stress management. Whether it's reading, gardening, art, or spending time in nature, these activities provide a reprieve from stressors and contribute to overall well-being.

Understanding the interconnectedness of stress and a healthy midsection highlights the importance of cultivating a holistic approach to well-being. Implementing stress management practices not only supports belly fat reduction but also contributes to enhanced resilience, emotional balance, and a more vibrant life.

Chapter 6

Recipes and Herbal Remedies

Healthy and Delicious Herbal Recipes

In the journey towards a flat tummy and overall well-being, the role of nutrition takes center stage. Incorporating herbal remedies into delicious and nutritious recipes not only enhances flavor but also provides a holistic approach to supporting digestive health. The following section explores a variety of healthy and delicious herbal recipes, showcasing the versatility of herbs in elevating the culinary experience while contributing to a flat tummy.

Herb-Infused Quinoa Salad:

Begin with a base of fluffy quinoa, a protein-rich grain that forms the foundation for this vibrant salad. Add a medley of fresh herbs such as parsley, cilantro, and mint to infuse the dish with a burst of flavor and nutritional benefits. Toss in colorful vegetables like cherry tomatoes, cucumber, and bell peppers for added crunch and vitamins. Dress the salad with a light vinaigrette featuring olive oil, lemon juice, and a touch of herbal favorites like oregano and thyme. This herb-infused quinoa salad not only satisfies the palate but also provides a nourishing option packed with essential nutrients.

Basil and Tomato Zoodle Bowl:
Embrace the trend of vegetable noodles, or "zoodles," by spiralizing zucchini to create a light and refreshing noodle alternative. In this recipe, the aromatic essence of basil takes center stage, enhancing the zoodles with its distinctive flavor. Toss the zoodles with cherry tomatoes, garlic, and a drizzle of olive oil. Finish the dish with a sprinkle of Parmesan cheese and a touch of fresh basil leaves. This low-carb and herb-centric zoodle bowl is not only visually appealing but also a delightful way to incorporate the benefits of basil into a satisfying meal.

Minty Watermelon and Feta Salad:
Harness the refreshing properties of mint in a summer-inspired watermelon and feta salad. Cube ripe watermelon and combine it with crumbled feta cheese for a sweet-and-savory contrast. The addition of chopped fresh mint leaves elevates the flavors and provides a cooling sensation. A drizzle of

balsamic glaze or a sprinkle of black pepper can enhance the taste further. This minty watermelon and feta salad offer a hydrating and herb-infused option that can be enjoyed as a light meal or a refreshing side dish.

Rosemary-Lemon Grilled Chicken:
Elevate grilled chicken with the aromatic combination of rosemary and lemon. Marinate chicken breasts with a mixture of fresh rosemary, minced garlic, lemon zest, and olive oil. Allow the flavors to meld before grilling to perfection. The result is a savory and herb-infused grilled chicken that pairs well with a variety of sides. Whether served with roasted vegetables, a quinoa salad, or a simple green salad, this rosemary-lemon grilled chicken adds a burst of herbal goodness to the protein component of a balanced meal.

These recipes showcase the versatility of herbs in enhancing the culinary experience while contributing to a flat tummy. Experimenting with different herb combinations allows individuals to tailor recipes to their preferences and nutritional needs. Whether seeking a light and refreshing salad, a flavorful zoodle bowl, or a savory grilled protein, incorporating herbs into everyday meals can be a delicious and health-conscious choice.

DIY Herbal Remedies for Flat Tummy

In addition to infusing herbs into culinary creations, do-it-yourself (DIY) herbal remedies offer a more direct and concentrated approach to leveraging the therapeutic properties of herbs for promoting a flat tummy. These remedies can be easily prepared at home, allowing individuals to take an active role in their wellness journey. The following section explores various DIY herbal remedies, each designed to address specific aspects of digestive health and contribute to achieving a flatter stomach.

Peppermint Infusion for Digestive Comfort:
Peppermint, with its menthol compound, is renowned for its ability to soothe the digestive tract and alleviate symptoms of indigestion, bloating, and gas. Creating a peppermint infusion is a simple yet effective DIY remedy. Steep a handful of fresh peppermint leaves or a teaspoon of dried peppermint in hot water. Allow it to infuse for several minutes, and then strain the leaves. The resulting peppermint infusion can be sipped after meals or during

moments of digestive discomfort to promote digestive comfort and reduce bloating.

Ginger-Lemon Elixir for Metabolism Boost:
Ginger, celebrated for its anti-inflammatory and metabolism-boosting properties, pairs seamlessly with the citrusy zing of lemon in a DIY elixir. Grate fresh ginger and combine it with freshly squeezed lemon juice in a glass of warm water. Optionally, add a drizzle of honey for sweetness. This ginger-lemon elixir serves as a revitalizing and invigorating drink that not only aids in digestion but also supports metabolic functions. Consuming it in the morning or before meals can be a refreshing ritual to kickstart the day.

Turmeric Golden Milk for Anti-Inflammatory Support:
Turmeric, prized for its active compound curcumin with anti-inflammatory properties, forms the basis of the well-known golden milk. In a saucepan, combine turmeric powder with coconut milk or any preferred milk alternative. Add a pinch of black pepper to enhance the absorption of curcumin. Sweeten the golden milk with a touch of honey or maple syrup, and heat the mixture until warm. This DIY turmeric

golden milk offers a comforting and anti-inflammatory beverage that can be enjoyed in the evening as a soothing bedtime ritual.

Fennel Seed Infusion for Digestive Ease:
Fennel seeds, known for their carminative properties that help alleviate gas and bloating, can be transformed into a digestive infusion. Crush a tablespoon of fennel seeds and steep them in hot water. Allow the seeds to infuse for about 10 minutes before straining. This fennel seed infusion can be consumed as a warm tea after meals to promote digestive ease. The mild licorice flavor adds a pleasant touch to the infusion, making it both soothing and beneficial for digestive health.

Cinnamon Honey Water for Blood Sugar Balance:
Cinnamon, with its potential to improve insulin sensitivity, can be incorporated into a DIY remedy to support blood sugar balance. Mix a teaspoon of cinnamon powder with warm water and add a teaspoon of honey for sweetness. Stir the mixture well and consume it regularly. This cinnamon honey water provides a flavorful and natural way to

incorporate the blood sugar-regulating properties of cinnamon into daily routines.

These DIY herbal remedies offer accessible and practical ways to harness the benefits of herbs for digestive health and a flat tummy. Integrating these remedies into daily routines allows individuals to take proactive steps in supporting their well-being. It's important to note that individual responses to herbs may vary, and consulting with healthcare professionals or herbalists is advisable, especially for those with pre-existing health conditions or concerns.

Incorporating Herbs into Everyday Meals

Beyond specific herbal recipes and remedies, seamlessly integrating herbs into everyday meals adds depth of flavor, nutritional benefits, and a touch of herbal goodness to a variety of dishes. This approach allows individuals to reap the rewards of herbs in a sustainable and enjoyable manner. Here are creative ways to incorporate herbs into everyday meals:

Herb-Infused Oils and Dressings:
Create herb-infused oils and dressings by combining fresh or dried herbs with olive oil or other preferred oils. Use these infused oils as a base for salad dressings, drizzle them over grilled vegetables, or incorporate them into marinades for meats. Basil, thyme, rosemary, and oregano are excellent choices for infusing oils, adding a burst of herbal flavor to various dishes.

Fresh Herbs in Soups and Stews:
Elevate the flavor profile of soups and stews by adding a handful of fresh herbs during the cooking process. Whether it's parsley in a chicken soup, cilantro in a lentil stew, or dill in a vegetable broth, fresh herbs contribute freshness and vibrancy to the dish. Consider adding herbs towards the end of the cooking time to preserve their delicate flavors.

Herb-Infused Waters and Iced Teas:
Stay hydrated with herb-infused waters or iced teas. Experiment with combinations like cucumber and mint, lemon and basil, or rosemary and berries. Allow the herbs to infuse in cold water or tea for a

refreshing beverage that not only quenches thirst but also provides a subtle herbal twist.

Herb Garnishes for Visual Appeal:
Enhance the visual appeal of dishes by using fresh herb garnishes. Sprinkle chopped cilantro over tacos, add a sprig of thyme to roasted vegetables, or scatter basil leaves on a caprese salad. Herb garnishes not only contribute to aesthetics but also offer a burst of flavor that elevates the overall dining experience.

Herbal Infusions in Grains and Legumes:
Infuse grains and legumes with herbal goodness by adding fresh or dried herbs during the cooking process. For example, stir chopped dill into cooked quinoa, toss rosemary into a pot of simmering lentils, or mix thyme with rice. This simple addition imparts herbal nuances to staple ingredients, transforming them into flavorful and aromatic components of a meal.

Incorporating herbs into everyday meals is a culinary adventure that adds both nutritional value and sensory delight. Whether through infusions, garnishes, or creative applications in cooking, herbs can become integral components of a well-rounded and flavorful diet. This approach allows individuals to effortlessly integrate the benefits of herbs into their culinary repertoire, contributing to both palate satisfaction and overall well-being.

Chapter 7

Maintaining Long-Term Results

Sustaining a flat tummy is not merely about short-term remedies; it involves establishing sustainable habits that contribute to overall well-being

Establishing Sustainable Habits

The foundation of maintaining long-term results lies in the establishment of sustainable habits that align with individual lifestyles and preferences. Crash diets or extreme workout regimens may offer quick fixes, but they often prove to be unsustainable in the long run. Sustainable habits, on the other hand, are those that can be seamlessly integrated into daily life, promoting consistency and gradual progress.

One key aspect of sustainable habits is the cultivation of a balanced and varied diet. Rather than adhering to restrictive diets, individuals can focus on incorporating nutrient-dense foods, including a diverse array of fruits, vegetables, whole grains, lean proteins, and healthy fats. Embracing moderation and mindfulness in eating fosters a healthy relationship with food and prevents the cycle of extreme restrictions followed by overindulgence.

Regular physical activity is another cornerstone of sustainable habits for maintaining a flat tummy. Instead of viewing exercise as a temporary effort to shed pounds, it should be embraced as a lifelong commitment to overall health. Finding enjoyable forms of exercise, whether it's walking, swimming, dancing, or practicing yoga, ensures that individuals are more likely to adhere to their fitness routines over the long term.

Adequate sleep and stress management also play crucial roles in sustaining positive outcomes. Prioritizing quality sleep supports overall well-being, including hormonal balance and metabolism. Stress, if left unmanaged, can contribute to the accumulation of visceral fat. Adopting stress-reducing practices such as mindfulness, meditation, or engaging in hobbies contributes to a more balanced and resilient approach to life.

Tracking Progress and Adjusting the Approach

Maintaining long-term results necessitates an awareness of progress and a willingness to adjust approaches based on individual responses. Tracking progress involves more than just monitoring weight; it encompasses various indicators such as changes in energy levels, mood, and overall well-being. Keeping a journal or using apps to record meals, exercise routines, and emotional states provides valuable insights into patterns and trends.

When tracking progress, it's essential to approach it with a holistic perspective. While visible changes in body composition are significant, non-scale victories such as improved digestion, increased energy, and enhanced mood should also be acknowledged. Celebrating these victories reinforces the positive impact of lifestyle changes and motivates individuals to stay committed to their long-term goals.

Adjusting the approach involves flexibility and adaptability. Bodies respond differently to various interventions, and what works for one person may not be suitable for another. If a particular exercise routine becomes monotonous or a dietary approach feels restrictive, it may be time to explore alternatives. The key is to listen to the body's signals and make adjustments that align with individual needs and preferences.

Periodic reassessment of goals is a valuable practice in maintaining long-term results. As individuals evolve, so do their priorities and aspirations. Adjusting goals to reflect changing circumstances ensures that the pursuit of a flat tummy remains relevant and aligned with overall well-being. Whether it involves setting new fitness challenges, exploring different types of physical activities, or fine-tuning dietary choices, adapting goals contributes to sustained motivation.

Herbal Maintenance for a Lasting Flat Tummy

Herbs, with their diverse therapeutic properties, can play a integral role in the maintenance of a lasting flat tummy. Integrating herbal maintenance involves incorporating herbs into daily routines to support digestive health, metabolism, and overall well-being. The following herbs are particularly noteworthy for their contributions to maintaining a flat tummy:

Fennel: Known for its carminative properties, fennel supports digestion and helps alleviate bloating. Drinking fennel tea after meals can be a simple and effective way to incorporate this herb into a daily routine.

Dandelion: Often used as a gentle diuretic, dandelion can aid in reducing water retention and supporting liver health. Dandelion tea or incorporating dandelion greens into salads are ways to benefit from this herbal ally.

Ginger: Renowned for its anti-inflammatory and digestive benefits, ginger can be consumed in various forms. Whether it's in tea, grated into dishes, or taken in supplement form, ginger supports digestive comfort and overall well-being.

Turmeric: The active compound curcumin in turmeric has anti-inflammatory properties. Including turmeric in cooking, making turmeric-infused golden milk, or taking turmeric supplements contributes to a healthy inflammatory response and supports digestive health.

Peppermint: With its menthol compound, peppermint helps relax the muscles of the gastrointestinal tract, reducing spasms and alleviating symptoms of indigestion. Peppermint tea or adding fresh peppermint leaves to dishes are delightful ways to enjoy this herb.

Cinnamon: Known for its potential to regulate blood sugar levels, cinnamon can be incorporated into various recipes. Sprinkling cinnamon on oatmeal, adding it to smoothies, or enjoying it in herbal infusions contributes to blood sugar balance.

Incorporating these herbs into daily life not only enhances the flavor of meals and beverages but also provides ongoing support for digestive health. Creating herbal routines, such as enjoying a cup of herbal tea after meals or experimenting with herbal-infused recipes, contributes to the overall maintenance of a flat tummy.

Conclusion

Embracing a healthier lifestyle is a transformative journey that extends beyond the pursuit of a flat tummy—it's a commitment to overall well-being and vitality. As you embark on this path, remember that every positive choice, no matter how small, contributes to a healthier and more fulfilling life.

Celebrate your victories, both seen and unseen. Whether it's the energy gained from a nourishing meal, the joy found in a favorite exercise routine, or the newfound sense of balance in managing stress, these are the building blocks of a healthier you. Recognize the journey as a series of steps, each one leading you closer to sustained well-being.

In moments of challenge, remember the resilience within you. Adjust your approach with kindness and understanding, acknowledging that growth often involves both progress and setbacks. Cultivate a mindset that values the journey as much as the destination, finding joy in the daily habits that contribute to a healthier and more vibrant life.

Surround yourself with a supportive community—whether friends, family, or like-minded individuals on a similar journey. Share experiences, seek encouragement, and offer support. The collective energy of a supportive network can be a powerful catalyst for positive change.

As you weave herbal remedies, nutritious choices, and mindful practices into your daily life, let them become integral parts of a holistic and sustainable lifestyle. Cherish the moments of self-care, savor the flavors of nourishing foods, and relish the invigorating benefits of movement. Allow these elements to not only contribute to a flat tummy but to shape a life rich in vitality and well-being.

Find encouragement to continue embracing the journey towards a healthier lifestyle—one that extends beyond physical appearance to encompass the holistic tapestry of your well-being. Your commitment to health is a gift to yourself, and with each intentional choice, you are sculpting a future filled with vitality, balance, and lasting wellness. May your path be filled with continued growth, self-love, and the flourishing rewards of a healthier, happier you.

www.ingramcontent.com/pod-product-compliance
Lightning Source LLC
Chambersburg PA
CBHW071056260726
48661CB00006B/2311